RECOVERY

A Physician's Unbelievable Story

RECOVERY

A Physician's Unbelievable Story

DANIEL ADEGOKE

Story Terrace

To my family and patients,
This memoir is dedicated to you—the heartbeats of my journey. To my family, who have been my fortress in the storm, your unwavering support has been my anchor in the toughest of times. And to my patients, whose bravery and resilience in the face of illness inspire me daily, you remind me why I chose this path. Together, you have shaped my story, teaching me the deepest lessons of love, perseverance, and hope. Thank you for standing by me and for trusting me to be part of your lives.

With all my love and gratitude,

Daniel Adegoke

CONTENTS

PROLOGUE

I remember the whole episode. People assume it would be patchy and hard to retell but I can talk about all of it. I can tell them what the mental health team said to me when I asked them to remove the communication equipment that was attached to the rear of my skull. They said they would look at it a little later. They wanted to make sure I was settled in and they were worried I was dehydrated. While I was explaining to them that the equipment was broadcasting my thoughts to the world, they simply nodded and checked my chart. Then they asked me for my postcode, my full name and my occupation.

'I'm an emergency doctor.'

That was the only time they stopped what they were doing. 'I am. I'm a qualified doctor.' And as the words came out of my mouth I saw the doubt flicker across their faces and then I saw some sadness. Even if they believed me I could see they didn't think I would practise medicine ever again. I looked at the ceiling of the secure mental health unit. There were a few small stains and a smoke detector. It was 2015 and I had no idea where my life was going to go next.

How had I got here? I asked myself before I fell into a fitful, erratic sleep.

CHAPTER 1: FLYING IN

The 2nd of January, 2005. That day will always be in my memory as the start of my new life. As the plane descended into Heathrow Airport, a mix of emotions hit me—nervousness, anticipation and a lot of possibility, as long as I worked hard. This was it. I had made it to the UK, the land of opportunity, bright lights and better prospects. There was more for me here than in my home country—Nigeria.

Stepping off the plane and breathing in that crisp winter air, I couldn't stop smiling, even as the chill nipped at my cheeks. My brother-in-law was waiting for me in Arrivals and he greeted me with a warm embrace and a huge grin. We chatted non-stop in the car, on the way to my sister's home. He was full of stories of his life in London, of the work culture and the tax system, and as he chatted I gazed out the window with my eyes fixed on the glistening lights illuminating the city streets.

It was all so different from home, where the lack of steady power had forced me to study for my high school exams by lantern light because our community transformer had blown up. I could vividly recall those sweltering nights hunched over my books, sweat trickling down my temples as I squinted to read my notes in the dim light. But now, here I was, zooming past the illuminated shop fronts and lit-up homes, allowing myself to imagine, just for a moment, that those hardships were firmly behind me and that a brighter future lay ahead.

My sister and her husband were generous hosts. They were happy to let me stay with them for as long as it took for me to find my footing. I was eager to start contributing, to make something of myself and not be a burden. But that proved harder than anticipated, with my visitor's visa status restricting my ability to work. Still, I tried, applying for every position I could, only to face rejection after rejection at the interview stage. It was disheartening, but I refused to let it get me down.

Then came a ray of hope. I had applied for a clinical attachment post at Darent Valley Hospital in Dartford, not really expecting anything to come of it. After all, they had made it quite clear there was an extensive waiting list and competition was ferocious for the limited positions. But sometimes life has a way of surprising you.

It was April when I got the phone call. I heard an unfamiliar voice on the other end of the line. The caller was from the Human Resources Department at Darent Valley. At first, I was sure there had been some mistake. No, she assured me, a place had opened up, and the team wanted to know if I would be keen to start. I could not stop myself from shouting slightly as I responded with an enthusiastic 'Yes!'

And just like that, I found myself striding through the entrance of Darent Valley Hospital to begin my first experience of life in the UK medical system. I was full of enthusiasm, and keen to make a good impression. I wanted to soak up every bit of knowledge that I could. I needn't have worried as I was placed under the guidance of three remarkable consultants—Mr Kika, a fellow Nigerian who understood all too well the challenges of navigating a new healthcare system, Dr J Thurston and Mr Kerur.

Mr Kika and Mr Kerur, in particular, took me under their wings and went out of their way to provide extra teaching and encouragement. They would pull me aside and guide me through different topics and procedures with easy patience. Mr Kika was always willing to share his expertise and was an invaluable support to a fresh-faced doctor like me, who was finding his way. I couldn't have asked for a better mentor.

My day-to-day clinical attachment involved observing doctors in substantive posts carry out their duties. I was allowed to take a patient's history (ask questions) but not permitted to examine them. I would present my cases to Mr Kerur or Mr Kika. They would then probe what I should do next in terms of examination and treatments for my patients.

Even with limited access to the patients, I was learning the ropes and the tricks of the trade in emergency medicine. Every patient interaction starts with ABCDE: Airway, Breathing, Circulation, Disability and Exposure. It wasn't long before I started dreaming of this approach in my sleep. It was drilled into me from day one by both Mr Kika and Mr Kerur and became the outline of my patient notes. I felt I was learning a lot with their guidance and mentorship.

CHAPTER 2: FROM DARENT VALLEY HOSPITAL TO UCLH AND LEARNING FROM PROF SINGER

My next position was a clinical attachment at University College London Hospital (UCLH) in orthopaedics and trauma. If I thought I had been impressed by the calibre of consultants at Darent Valley, UCLH was about to set a whole new standard. I had the extraordinary good fortune of learning under Mr Johan Witt, a world-renowned orthopaedic surgeon whose reputation for excellence preceded him. He was a master and I watched closely as he performed complex procedures with calm and careful precision.

More than just a skilled technician, Mr Witt was also a natural teacher as he was always ready with a pearl of wisdom or a word of encouragement. Under his tutelage, I gained not only a deeper understanding of surgical techniques but valuable insights into holistic patient care. He emphasised the importance of seeing the person, not just the condition—a philosophy I carry with me to this day.

But as October 2006 drew to a close, so too did my opportunity with Mr Witt and then came the headache of renewing my visa. At the time, the requirements for doctors were changing and the process was becoming more convoluted. In short, I needed a job, and I needed one that could sponsor my visa and I had very little time to get it. It was a daunting prospect and if I could not find a solution I would have to return to Nigeria.

In those moments of uncertainty, I always found my thoughts turning to home to my family and the upbringing that had shaped me. I grew up in Nigeria to the sound of my many siblings playing, arguing, cooking and making plans for the future. I was one of eight children so I was used to a busy house where my older siblings would talk about their dreams. My parents had a strong work ethic and were often away so my grandmother would come to our house to take over our care. Even now, if I close my eyes tight enough, I can see her twinkling eyes and her sense of fun. She let us all get away with a lot more than our parents would ever have done and she loved us all so much.

When I was a child, I took after my mother who was a nurse and had a keen interest in science and medicine. She inspired me to become a doctor and I used to play with her stethoscope when I was about six or seven years old. This was something she encouraged and I often thought of her dedication to her patients when I was on the wards. Watching her care for others had first sparked my interest in medicine. I had many memories of her tending to the sick and suffering with such compassion that I would stop and watch knowing, deep in my bones, that this was what I wanted to do with my life.

I also thought of my father who headed a government parastatal offering technical advice and support to cocoa farmers in the South West region of Nigeria. He was a hard-working man, he had a large family to care for and he was often away from home. He had shown me the value of perseverance, of having your own goals and making sure you put your heart and soul into something you believed in.

With family love and support to bolster me, I knew I could weather whatever storms came my way. I had come too far to give up now. So I redoubled my efforts to find a way to stay in the UK and continue pursuing my dreams. It wouldn't be easy, but then again, nothing worthwhile ever is.

Fortunately, just before my visa expired, Darent Valley Hospital offered me the position of Senior House Officer in Emergency Medicine. It was for one year and it was tough but I learned a great deal. My shifts usually started around 5 p.m. and finished around 2 a.m. This schedule wasn't ideal for learning from senior doctors who typically finished work as I arrived so I began to feel frustrated that I could be learning more. Nonetheless, I persevered, gained experience and dealt with my frustrations.

The year flew by as I spent the bulk of my time in the fast-paced world of emergency medicine, always impressed by the talent and dedication of the team that treated the stream of patients coming through the doors. It was exhausting, demanding, exhilarating and everything I had hoped it would be.

Thirteen months at Darent Valley had zipped past but I was staring at my visa expiration date once again, seriously worried about being able to stay. But at the ninth hour, the phone rang and a Registrar position at the Emergency

Department at UCLH had come up. I got the role and worked there from November 2007 until April 2010, gaining further experience and honing my emergency medicine skills. In April 2010, an opportunity arose for a four-month secondment to the intensive care unit (ICU) This was perfect as it allowed me to complete my rotation and gain critical care experience as part of my emergency medicine training.

It was during this secondment that I met Professor Mervyn Singer, a pivotal figure who would shape my medical career aspirations. Professor Singer embodied everything I aspired to be as a doctor—immensely knowledgeable, dedicated to teaching, and approachable to his staff and students.

From our first interactions, Professor Singer took an interest in nurturing my development. He was the first one to plant the seed of pursuing a PhD and becoming an expert in a particular medical field. His teaching style was engaging and he gave me autonomy to assess patients under his guidance, demonstrating a trust in my abilities that boosted my confidence.

I felt inspired watching Professor Singer interact with the medical team. His depth of knowledge was astounding and he always made himself available to thoroughly explain conditions and treatment plans. He would call on us to answer questions and make sure we were truly learning in a hands-on way as we worked alongside him. The rounds may have taken longer with his meticulous teaching style, but we gained so much from the extra time he gave us all.

Professor Singer's mentorship had a huge impact on my desire to pursue research and teaching in my own career. He made me feel like a valued member of the team, even though I was joining the ICU from the Emergency Department. There was never a sense that I was out of my depth—he welcomed my perspectives and contributions.

After four rewarding months, I had to return to the Emergency Department as they were still funding my position. I would have relished the opportunity to stay longer in the ICU learning from Professor Singer. However, I carried the lessons and influence from my time with him as I progressed in my emergency medicine training.

Back in the Emergency Department, I continued working on my competencies and documentation needed for the Certificate of Eligibility for Specialist Registration (CESR) pathway. This alternative route to achieving specialist registration in the UK is less defined than the formal training pathway. It requires more self-direction and diligence to ensure all the necessary competencies are met and signed off by consultants.

At this stage in my career, I had no idea how arduous pursuing the CESR pathway would make my professional journey as it lacks formal structure and the very subjective nature of it is daunting. I felt unsupported and unprepared to navigate such a poorly defined path to becoming a consultant.

I had survived the demands of medical school and even that had not equipped me to deal with the CESR training route. The seven years I spent at the College of Medicine, University of Ibadan in Nigeria had been tough. There were countless exams and hoops to jump through on the path to adding the title of 'Dr' to my name but I had achieved it.

I vividly remember the anxiety and then elation I felt after passing the First MB exam, the one that determined whether you moved from the non-clinical to clinical years and could continue in medical school. Around half of my classmates had failed that crucial exam. When the results were posted, I wasn't even at the school—the tension was too much and I stayed at home in Ibadan, waiting for news. My good friend Dr Ajibade, who I called Dotun, phoned to tell me I had passed. The relief I felt at that moment was indescribable as the thought of repeating all the studying would have been hard for me to do.

My family had always considered me brilliant, perhaps even a genius. But after struggling through the challenges of medical school alongside so many other bright minds, I gained a new perspective. In an environment where everyone is brilliant, what distinguishes those who succeed is primarily their endurance and resilience. The First MB exam was just one of many challenges that tested those qualities and foreshadowed the uncertainties I would face in my medical career.

Now on the uncertain CESR pathway, I once again found myself needing to muster that resilience to forge ahead on an undefined path. My professional life was now rife with subjectivity and lacking clear goalposts. I had never felt so adrift in my career, and I wonder sometimes if this was starting to affect me. After conquering the hurdles of medical school and beginning what I thought would be a reasonably straightforward path to becoming a consultant in emergency medicine, I now felt thrust into a strange sort of limbo, unsure of my next steps.

I knew I had to persevere, relying on the same determination that had seen me through relentless exams and other challenges. I threw myself into my work, continuing to develop my skills in the Emergency Department while seeking out opportunities to gain the needed competencies for my CESR portfolio. Even with the monumental challenge ahead of me, giving up was not an option. I decided to work harder than ever to prove myself.

CHAPTER 3: MEETING DR BROWN

February 2011 marked a significant transition in my medical career as I bid farewell to UCLH and embarked on a new chapter at St Mary's Hospital in Paddington. My time at UCLH had given me confidence in my skills in emergency medicine and intensive care treatment. However, I knew that to continue growing as a clinician and reach my ultimate goal of becoming a consultant, I needed to seek out fresh challenges and learn from a diverse range of experts in my field.

One of the key factors that drew me to St Mary's was the opportunity to work with Dr Ruth Brown, a renowned figure who held the position of Vice President (Academics) for the Royal College of Emergency Medicine. I had heard about her reputation as a brilliant clinician and a passionate advocate for excellence in emergency care. I hoped that under her guidance, I would gain invaluable insights into the intricacies of the speciality and navigate the complex path towards becoming a consultant.

My journey at St Mary's began in the Paediatric Emergency Department. It was an incredibly busy unit. There was a constant influx of young patients presenting with a wide range of conditions, from minor injuries to life-threatening illnesses. The unpredictable nature of paediatric emergencies meant that we had to be prepared for anything, at any time, all of the time!

I quickly learned that working in paediatric emergency medicine required a unique set of skills and a deep understanding of the specific needs of children. Unlike adults, children often struggle to articulate their symptoms clearly, and their vital signs can deteriorate rapidly if not closely monitored. It was crucial to develop a keen eye for subtle signs of distress and to communicate effectively with both the young patients and their anxious parents.

One of the biggest challenges I faced during my time in the Paediatric Emergency Department was the high patient volume, particularly during night shifts when fewer doctors were on duty. It was not uncommon for me to be the only registrar on the floor, tasked with overseeing the entire department and making critical decisions about patient care. Although I had the support of the paediatric team, the pressure to manage multiple cases simultaneously while ensuring the highest standards of care was immense.

Despite the demanding nature of the work, I found my time in paediatric emergency medicine to be incredibly rewarding. Seeing a child recover from a serious illness or injury and watching the relief on their parents' faces reminded me of why I had chosen this path. It was a privilege to be able to make a difference in the lives of these young patients and their families.

After five intense months in the Paediatric Emergency Department, I transitioned to the Adult Emergency Department at St Mary's. I knew I would cross paths with Dr

Ruth Brown, and I was keen to meet her but our first meeting did not really go to plan.

In fact, most of my first interactions with Dr Brown were far from smooth. During a case review session, she highlighted a case I had managed involving a patient with chronic obstructive pulmonary disease and heart failure who was admitted with a suspected heart attack. Dr Brown meticulously scrutinised every step of my management plan, from the initial assessment to the decision to refer the patient to the medical team.

As I stood there, defending my actions and my clinical reasoning, I could feel the weight of Dr Brown's gaze upon me. She had a reputation for being a tough but fair critic, and I knew that every decision I had made would be dissected and analysed. It was a nerve-wracking experience, and I could feel my anxiety levels rising as I tried to justify everything I had done for the patient.

However, as the discussion progressed, I began to appreciate the depth of Dr Brown's knowledge and her unwavering commitment to patient safety. She posed challenging questions and pushed me to consider alternative approaches, always with the goal of providing the best possible care for our patients. It was clear that she had incredibly high expectations for her team, and she was not afraid to hold us accountable for our decisions.

Over time, I came to understand that Dr Brown's intensity and attention to detail were not meant to intimidate or belittle, but rather to inspire us to strive for excellence in everything we did. She had an uncanny ability to know everything that was happening in the department at any given moment, from the number of patients waiting to be seen to the status of each ongoing case. To this day I have no idea how she managed to have an eye on everything as well as complete her own work. Her dedication was unparalleled, and she led by example, often seeing patients herself when the department was particularly busy.

Working with Dr Brown changed me. She wanted us to be the best and she showed us how to be personally and professionally excellent. She taught me the importance of thorough clinical reasoning, effective communication and meticulous attention to detail. Under her guidance, I learned to anticipate potential complications, to think critically about each case, and to always prioritise patient safety above all else.

One particular skill that she taught me was the value of asking for feedback and learning from constructive criticism. Dr Brown was never afraid to point out areas where I could improve, but she always did so in a way that was supportive and encouraging. She recognised potential in me that I had not yet seen in myself, and she challenged me to rise to the occasion and become the best doctor I could be.

As I reflect on my time working with Dr Brown, I am filled with a deep sense of gratitude for the lessons she imparted and the mentorship she provided. While our relationship may have gotten off to a rocky start, I came to appreciate her as not just a colleague, but as a role model and a guiding force in my career. Her dedication to her patients, her commitment to lifelong learning, and her tireless efforts to advance the field of emergency medicine continue to inspire me to this day. Now I think about it, Dr Brown's standards were similar to my mother's when she was nursing. If they had ever worked together they would have made a great team.

In September 2012, after an intense period of learning and growth at St Mary's, I made the decision to take a break from the hospital to gain experience in acute medicine and anaesthetics. These rotations are essential requirements for emergency medicine training in the UK, and I knew that they would provide me with valuable skills and knowledge I could apply in my future practice.

My first stop was UCLH, where I spent four months from October 2012 to February 2013 immersed in the world of acute medicine. While it was certainly an educational experience, I found myself missing the fast-paced, adrenaline-fuelled environment of the Emergency Department.

In acute medicine, most of the patients I encountered had already been stabilised by the emergency team, and my role was primarily to continue their care and manage their ongoing treatment. I had the opportunity to delve deeper into the management of complex medical conditions but I couldn't shake the feeling that something was missing. I longed for the unpredictability and the sense of immediacy that came with working in emergency medicine, where every moment counted and every decision had the potential to save a life.

After four months in acute medicine, I knew that it was time to move on. While I was grateful for the experience and the knowledge I had gained, my heart was firmly rooted in emergency medicine. I made the decision to leave UCLH and embark on the next stage of my training: anaesthetics.

Securing a standalone anaesthetics position in London was much tougher than I had anticipated. Most of the available posts were embedded within formal training programs, which meant that they were not accessible to doctors like myself who were pursuing an alternative route to specialist registration. Faced with limited options in the capital, I made the practical decision to look further afield.

In 2013 I found myself heading to Scunthorpe General Hospital for my anaesthesia rotation. It was a big change from the bustling streets of London and the familiar halls of UCLH and St Mary's, but I was determined to make the most of the experience. After all, I needed specific skills to become a well-rounded emergency medicine specialist.

I had no idea that this simple decision, driven by the practical realities of my training pathway, would forever alter the course of my life. As I packed my bags and prepared for the move to Scunthorpe, I had no idea of what lay ahead for me. I was about to go through a period that would have an enormous impact on my personal and professional journey.

I settled into my flat in Barton-upon-Humber (about 20 minutes from Scunthorpe) and I couldn't help but reflect on the path that had led me to this point. My mind wandered back to my early years, to the experiences that had shaped me and set me on the course towards a career in medicine.

I vividly remembered my time at Oritamefa Baptist Model School, the private primary school where I spent six formative years. Most of my memories from that period are sweet and carefree, but there was one aspect of school life that I dreaded: getting dressed for school in the morning. It was a daily struggle. I simply wanted to stay in the comfort of my pyjamas, while my parents were adamant that I should get dressed and go to school! But despite the battle of wills in the mornings, my childhood was a happy one. As one of the younger children of several siblings, my needs were always taken care of, and my only real source of stress was competing for my parents' attention. Academically, I excelled, consistently ranking among the top five students in my class. Life, it seemed, couldn't get any better.

That had all changed when I passed the entrance exams for Government College Ibadan, a prestigious public secondary school for boys. Excited by the prospect of this new chapter in my life, I enrolled as a boarding student for my first year. Little did I know that this decision would lead to one of the most challenging periods of my young life.

The transition from the sheltered world of private primary school to the harsh realities of a public boarding school was a shock to my system. I found myself at the mercy of older students who subjected me to relentless bullying and forced me to perform various forms of hard labour, from cutting grass to cleaning toilets. It was a far cry from the carefree days of my childhood, and I quickly realised that I was not cut out for this new, uncomfortable way of life.

Desperate to escape the torment of boarding school, I poured my heart out in letters to my parents, pleading with them to allow me to return home. After a year of enduring the hardships of boarding life, my parents finally relented, but not without a stern warning: if my grades were to slip, I would be sent back to the boarding house.

Motivated by fear and a determination to never again experience the horrors of my first year, I threw myself into my studies with a renewed sense of purpose. Over the next six years, I consistently came first in all of my subjects, earning scholarships that covered my school fees and cementing my place at the top of my class. It was a hard-fought victory, a testament to my resilience and my ability to adapt when the pressure was upon me.

As I sat in my new accommodation in Barton-upon-Humber, surrounded by the unfamiliar sights and sounds of a new town, I couldn't help but draw parallels between my childhood experiences and the challenges I now faced as a doctor in training. Just as I had navigated the transition from primary to secondary school, I knew that I would need to draw upon my inner strength and adaptability to succeed in this new phase of my life.

CHAPTER 4: A TEST OF RESILIENCE—THE SCUNTHORPE INCIDENT AND AFTERMATH

Scunthorpe General Hospital's Anaesthesia Department was very different from the welcoming environment I had experienced in London. On my first day, I walked in and instantly felt like an outsider. The team referred to me as a novice, despite my years of experience in emergency medicine. The consultants had their own way of doing things and I tried my best to fit in, but there was an unspoken tension, a sense that I didn't quite belong. I found I was reluctant when I got dressed in the mornings but I still went in on time and remained professional.

Dr Kumar was the exception. He was a knowledgeable consultant who could teach for hours, patiently explaining concepts and guiding me through procedures. I enjoyed working with him immensely. However, not everyone shared his open and collaborative approach.

One consultant in particular seemed to take issue with me from the start. In his eyes, I believe I came across as too confident, too sure of myself. Perhaps it was my London training or the fact that I wasn't afraid to ask questions and challenge the status quo. 'Why are we doing what we're doing?' I would inquire. 'Is there an evidence base for it?' My curiosity and desire to understand was met with disapproval rather than encouragement.

Despite these undercurrents, I earned my Initial Assessment of Competence certificate after three months, allowing me to take on more responsibility. I started doing on-calls and night shifts managing ICU patients. It was demanding work, but I enjoyed the challenge and the opportunity to make a difference.

On one fateful evening, I was called to the ICU to see if any patients needed my attention. A senior colleague, a registrar, mentioned that a central line needed to be inserted and asked if I wanted to do the procedure under his supervision. I readily agreed—it would be my first time performing a central line independently at Scunthorpe, but I had done it many times before and was totally comfortable with the procedure.

We prepared the patient, deepening their sedation with propofol. I carefully inserted the needle into the neck, threading the guide wire through once I was certain I was in the correct position. Using the ultrasound probe, I double-checked the guide-wire placement. Everything looked perfect.

Just as I set down the probe to continue the procedure, a shout rang out from the end of the room. 'Stop! What are you doing?'

Startled, I looked up to see the disapproving consultant striding towards me, his face a mask of anger. I explained that I was putting in a central line under the registrar's supervision, but he demanded to see for himself. I picked up the probe again and showed him the guide wire was exactly where it should be. Seeing this, he seemed to relax slightly and moved away to join the nurses' station.

But the damage was done. His sudden interruption had broken my concentration at a crucial moment. As I went to continue, I realised my hand, slick with ultrasound gel, had lost its grip on the delicate wire. To my horror, I felt it slip from my grasp and disappear into the patient's vascular system.

'I've lost the guide wire,' I called out, my voice shaking. The consultant rushed back over and together we located the wayward wire on ultrasound. It had migrated dangerously far, coming to rest in one of the heart's ventricles.

What followed was a whirlwind of activity as we arranged for an emergency transfer to Hull Royal Infirmary's Interventional Radiology Department. I rode in the ambulance with the patient, my heart in my throat the entire journey. The radiologists were ready and waiting when we arrived, and they skillfully removed the guide wire via catheter through the femoral vein. I could finally breathe again when they declared it a success. We transported the stable patient back to Scunthorpe, and I headed home for the night, completely drained by the events.

The incident weighed heavily on my mind over the following days and weeks. I knew there would be an investigation, a root cause analysis to determine what went wrong and how to prevent it from happening again. I naively believed it would be an objective process, a collaborative effort to identify any failings in the system and make positive changes.

Instead, what I walked into felt more like an ambush. The focus was solely on my actions, with barely a mention of the consultant's untimely and disruptive intervention. 'It looks like you're not competent enough, that's why this happened,' they concluded, their words like a punch to the gut. I tried to defend myself, to plead my case, but it was clear the decision had already been made.

In the aftermath, the Head of Department took me aside. 'These things happen,' he said, not unkindly. 'You just need to do more central lines under supervision, get signed off properly.'

I nodded numbly, but inside I was reeling. How could they not see that the consultant's actions had directly contributed to the error? Why was I the only one being held accountable? The injustice of it burnt like acid in my throat.

Still, I tried to take the advice on board, to use the incident as a learning opportunity. But something had shifted inside me. The confidence and enthusiasm I once had were shattered, replaced by a gnawing self-doubt that coloured everything I did. I second-guessed every decision and lay awake at night replaying each interaction, each procedure, looking for flaws and mistakes.

My appetite vanished and I could barely force myself to eat. Sleep was even more elusive, my mind constantly whirring with anxious thoughts. For two long months, I struggled on, throwing myself into my work in an attempt to prove myself, to regain the trust and respect I was sure I had lost.

But the damage ran too deep. By October 2013, three months after that fateful day, I could no longer ignore the toll it was taking on my mental and physical health. With a heavy heart, I submitted my resignation.

I remained in my little Barton-upon-Humber flat for nearly three months. During that time it hit me just how much pressure I had been under, how close I was to cracking. I had no way of knowing then how fragile I would soon become, how the cracks that incident created would spread and deepen until I could barely hold myself together.

CHAPTER 5: LOSING EVERYTHING THAT WAS REAL

The incident at Scunthorpe General Hospital had shaken me to my core. In the months that followed, I found myself slipping into a dark abyss, my mind consumed by thoughts of failure and inadequacy.

At first, I brushed off the symptoms as exhaustion and stress. The long hours, the demanding cases, the constant pressure to perform—it was all part of the job, I told myself. But as the weeks turned into months, I could no longer ignore the warning signs.

Sleep became rare, my nights were haunted by vivid nightmares and going over and over what had happened. Food lost its appeal, and I found myself eating occasionally as my appetite had vanished along with my sense of purpose. A heaviness settled over me, a blanket of nothingness that seemed to drain the colour from the world.

I retreated from everything and remained isolated in my Barton-upon-Humber flat. For two long months, I barely left the house, shutting out the concerned calls and messages from loved ones. It was as if I had pressed pause on every part of my life.

When I finally mustered the strength to return to London in December 2013, I hoped that the familiar surroundings and the support of my sister would be enough to pull me up.

Being with my family had always been the secret of my success. I threw myself back into work, taking on locum shifts and trying to regain some sense of normality.

But everything was not the same. I was still seriously down. In February 2014, I found myself back at St Mary's Hospital, working under the guidance of Dr Ruth Brown. Despite her warm welcome and the familiarity of the department, I couldn't shake the feeling that something was terribly wrong.

It started with a nagging sense of unease, a prickling at the back of my neck that made me feel like I was being watched. One morning I was with a patient and I was sure that he was not genuine. His description of his problems sounded as if he had read them from the internet. The next patient behaved in the same way and I became convinced that the people I was seeing were not real. I was sure that they were actors sent to test my knowledge and report back to my superiors on my failings. This seemed a reasonable way to test me in case anyone thought I might make a mistake again. It became impossible to focus on my work.

I decided to confide in Dr Brown, hoping that she may also have had actors sent to her at some point in her career. Always professional, she listened patiently as I poured out my fears and she took them seriously. She reached out to her colleagues at UCLH, trying to determine if actors were in the hospital and if there was any truth to my suspicions.

'Daniel,' she said gently, 'I've spoken with everyone in the department, and I can assure you that no one is sending actors to test you. The patients you've been seeing are genuine, and your work has been exemplary.'

Her words should have been a comfort, but they only served to deepen my confusion. If what she said was true, then what was happening to me? Why couldn't I trust my own perceptions?

The paranoia and delusions continued to escalate until I could no longer bear the weight of my own mind. I was referred to the occupational health team and after two appointments they concluded that they could not find anything wrong with me. This did not help me at all. Their conclusion heightened my paranoia to an extreme level. I was convinced that there was something seriously wrong with me and that the entire hospital was keeping it from me.

I decided my only option was to resign from my position. I handed my resignation letter to Dr Brown and decided to take on locum work which was mostly at Whittington Hospital. I think I was too busy at this time to realise how paranoid I had become but one night when the patients were sleeping and the other staff were on a break I heard someone talking to me. I turned around and there was no one with me but the voice was still clear as a bell. Even in my troubled state, I knew the voices had to be coming from me.

I finished dealing with my paperwork while this new and alien voice spoke to me constantly then I got into my car and drove straight to St Mary's Hospital and asked for Dr Ward.

'I'm hearing voices,' I confessed, my voice barely above a whisper. 'I don't know what's real anymore.'

Dr Ward listened to my story. Without hesitation, she referred me to a psychiatrist for assessment which I agreed to readily. But when the diagnosis came in, it was like a punch to the gut: *psychosis*. The word rang in my ears, a death knell for the life I had once known. How could I possibly continue my work as a doctor, responsible for the lives of others, when I couldn't even trust my own mind? It was over. Everything I had worked for was gone with that one word.

I was referred to community mental health services, but I had lost all self-awareness. I could not rationally analyse the state of my mental health now which meant I could not engage with anything they said to me. The St. Mary's psychiatrist reviewed me and sent a letter to my GP but by the time the GP wrote to me with a treatment plan I had had more terrible news. My sister contacted me to tell me that my father was very ill. My only thoughts were to be with him and give him medical care.

My friend, Dr Ajibade, was a rare beacon of light in those dark days. He encouraged me to prioritise my mental health above all else, to take the time I needed to heal and find my way back to myself.

'Your well-being is the most important thing,' he insisted, his voice firm but kind. 'Everything else can wait.'

But even as I struggled to come to terms with my new reality, life had other plans. In June 2014, I received word that my father wasn't doing well in Nigeria. Without a second thought, I booked a flight, my own troubles temporarily forgotten in the face of this new crisis.

For two weeks, I sat by my father's bedside, holding his hand and praying for a miracle. But despite my best efforts, his condition only worsened, and I was forced to return to the UK to deal with my mental health issues, the GMC and the medical processes in the NHS. I flew back to Heathrow but this time my heart was heavy with worry and guilt.

July brought more devastating news. My father passed away while I was in London. The grief was like a physical pain, a gaping wound that refused to heal. I cried as I had never cried before. I missed him so much.

As if the loss of my father wasn't enough, I received a letter from the GMC informing me of an investigation into my ability to practice medicine. The rest of my family advised me that travelling to Nigeria in September to bury my father was the right decision and that I should use that time to mourn but I was terrified that this meant losing my career altogether. In losing my Dad, I felt that I had lost everything I held dear in life. I was in so much pain that I began to wish I had died with him.

I returned to the UK on 29th September 2014 to attend the Interim Orders Panel hearing, my mind in complete turmoil. As I tried to explain my experiences to the panel, the words tumbled out in a jumbled mess.

'I believe I'm doing special work commissioned by God,' I rambled, my eyes wide and desperate. 'I have equipment in my brain that allows me to communicate with government operatives.'

The panel's decision was swift and merciless. My medical license was suspended pending further investigation. I would be required to see two GMC-appointed psychiatrists for assessment, their reports determining my fate. The decision felt like an ending to me. What was I going to do now?

In the months that followed, I sank deeper into despair. The loss of my father, combined with the unravelling of my career and the grip of psychosis, was too much for me to cope with. I had no one to guide me through the grieving process, no one to help me make sense of the chaos in my mind.

Growing up, I had always been taught that family was everything. As the sixth of eight children, I had never felt the pressure of being the firstborn or the indulgence of being the baby. Instead, I had revelled in the love and support of my siblings, secure in the knowledge that we would always be there for each other. I had always known that this was a gift.

But now, thousands of miles away from home and drowning, I missed my father beyond measure. The demands of working in the NHS, particularly in emergency care, had left little time for visits home or quality time with my dad. I had missed so much time with him.

The image of my once strong and vibrant father, reduced to a wheelchair and then to a bed, haunted me. I should have been there more, should have made the time to cherish the moments we had left. Instead, I had been consumed by exams, training and schedules unaware of precious time slipping away.

However, there was a saving grace amidst all the guilt and regret. My father, in a stubborn act of love and determination, had made one last trip in his wheelchair to visit his children in the UK in October 2011. He then travelled on to see my brother in the US before his health deteriorated to the point where he could no longer take trips abroad. It was a bittersweet memory, a reminder of the unbreakable bonds of family, even in the face of distance and hardship.

But still, I couldn't shake the feeling that I hadn't done enough, that I hadn't taken enough journeys home to be with him in his final years. The sacrifices I had made for my career suddenly seemed so small in comparison to the time I had lost with my father.

As I lay in bed at night, the weight of my regrets pressing down on my chest, I couldn't help but wonder what might have been different if I had made other choices. If I hadn't gone to Scunthorpe; if I had been more attentive to my own mental health; if I had been a better son and brother.

But the past was set in stone, and all I could do now was try to pick up the pieces of my shattered life. I knew that the road ahead would be long and difficult, that I would have to fight tooth and nail to reclaim my career, if that was even possible. And yet, even in the depths of my despair, a tiny ember of hope still flickered. I was a good doctor, a skilled and compassionate healer. I had worked too hard and come too far to let it all slip away.

So I made a promise to myself—I would do whatever it took to get well, to prove to myself and to the world that I was more than my diagnosis. I would lean on the love and support of my family, even from a distance, and I would honour my father's memory by living a life he would be proud of.

CHAPTER 6: THE ROAD TO RECOVERY AND REBUILDING MY LIFE

By June 2015, I was not in a better place. My psychotic symptoms had reached a breaking point. I was staying with my sister-in-law in Thamesmead, and my behaviour had become increasingly erratic. My sister and my dear friend, Dr Ajibade, recognised the severity of my condition and reached out for help. A psychiatric liaison nurse was sent to assess me, and after a thorough evaluation, the decision was made to section me under the Mental Health Act.

I was taken to the Queen Elizabeth Hospital in Woolwich and admitted to the psychiatric ward. The experience was surreal and disorienting, as I grappled with the realisation that I had lost control over my own life. After just a day or two, I was transferred to Cygnet Hospital in Blackheath, a secure psychiatric unit, due to the lack of available beds in Woolwich.

The month I spent at Cygnet Hospital was a turning point in my journey. I received oral medication, but the effects were slow to take hold. As I began to regain some clarity, I contested my involuntary hospitalisation, believing that I was well enough to return home. However, my appeal was denied by a tribunal panel, and I was forced to confront my new reality.

In the summer of 2015, I was transferred to Maidstone Hospital's psychiatric ward for another month of treatment. It was during this time that I began to gain insight into my condition and the critical role that medication played in managing my symptoms. I worked closely with the mental health team, learning about my illness and developing strategies for coping with the challenges ahead.

By the end of August 2015, I had made sufficient progress to be discharged from the hospital.

I was relieved to be returning to my life, but there was a problem. The medication I had been given was 10 mg of olanzapine to be taken in the morning and this drug has a tranquillising effect. I was so tired, I was sleeping a great deal during the day, so I could not see a way back to work. I was a doctor. That was my life. It was how I earned my living so I made the decision to leave the meds in my bathroom cabinet and continue with my career. It was a logical decision but it was a terrible mistake and I would lose everything because of it.

I had no idea how bad my financial position had become. As I moved into independent accommodation in Maidstone, I knew that I had to start rebuilding my life from the ground up.

I began working as a care worker, a job that allowed me to test my ability to manage stress and regain a sense of purpose. The work was challenging, with low pay, long hours and the demands of caring for patients with complex needs, such as dementia. Despite the difficulties, I found inspiration in the people around me, who worked tirelessly to provide compassionate care to vulnerable individuals.

Throughout this period, I continued to engage with community mental health services and attend GMC hearings regarding my fitness to practise. The process was emotionally draining, but I remained committed to demonstrating my ability to return to medicine.

In June 2017, I experienced a significant setback when I suffered a relapse of psychotic symptoms shortly after moving into a new apartment in Hayes. I made the difficult decision to voluntarily admit myself to a psychiatric unit for a month-long stay. During this time, my medication was refined, and a robust relapse prevention plan was put in place.

Upon discharge, I faced the added challenge of substantial rent arrears and the need to urgently vacate the apartment. With few options available, I relocated to a smaller, more affordable room in Bromley and focused on rebuilding my life once again, one step at a time.

The financial toll of my mental health struggles became increasingly apparent. In February 2017, I made the difficult decision to declare bankruptcy due to the accumulated debts and my inability to work during hospitalisations. The unpaid debts, totalling around £27,000, weighed heavily on my mind, but I knew that I had to take this step to move forward. I needed to be free from some of my stress and this seemed the easiest option to my exhausted mind.

Relocating to a smaller, more affordable room in Bromley, I focused on rebuilding once more. I had no choice. It was a slow process, a series of tiny steps forward punctuated by the occasional stumble. But I refused to give up, to let the setbacks define me. I just needed to get back on my path.

I found solace in the support of my loved ones, in the knowledge that I was not alone in my struggle. My family, though separated by distance, remained a constant source of strength and encouragement. And my friends, like the ever-loyal Dr Ajibade, stood by me through thick and thin.

As the weeks turned into months, I began to see glimmers of hope on the horizon. The care work, though challenging, provided a sense of purpose and structure to my days.

Slowly but surely, the confident and driven Daniel started to resurface. It was a gradual process, a delicate dance of two steps forward and one step back. But with each passing day, I felt a little stronger, a little more capable of facing the challenges ahead.

I recalled another time in my life that I had stayed in hospital. When I was at school I contracted pneumonia. I was seriously ill and had to be admitted to hospital. The treatment at that time was for me to have intramuscular antibiotics administered to the buttocks for 10 days. The injection was unbelievably painful and each time I had it I vowed to myself that I should work in medicine purely to stop treatments like the one I was subjected to. I felt that no human should have to feel so much pain in order to feel better. It did not make sense to me and even after I was discharged I found it hard to sit down or be comfortable for a further two weeks.

I replayed my memories of that time and I knew I just had to take the treatment and get out of the other side but I did not know if I was strong enough to do what I needed to do.

CHAPTER 7: TRIUMPH AND TRANSFORMATION—MY RETURN TO MEDICINE

My diagnosis was paranoid schizophrenia. This condition needs daily medication that can sometimes slow the patient down. To return to my beloved career in medicine seemed like an impossible dream. However, armed with newfound determination and the unwavering support of key allies, I decided I would at least try to reclaim my life despite all the advice I was being given.

Following my hospitalisation and my relapse, I continued to attend GMC hearings and work closely with my legal team to present evidence of my progress and mental stability. These hearings were nerve-wracking, as my entire livelihood and identity hung in the balance. However, I knew I had to carry on and advocate for myself if I wanted any chance of practising medicine again.

Throughout this period, I received heartening support from colleagues who believed in me. Dr Ruth Brown provided a letter attesting to my good character and capacity to return to practice. Her endorsement meant the world to me and fighting for my dream suddenly felt possible.

A pivotal moment arrived in August 2018 when I attended a crucial GMC hearing to present my case for returning to medical practice with appropriate supervision and monitoring. In the months leading up to the hearing, I poured myself into preparation, gathering evidence and rehearsing my arguments. I knew I had to convince the panel that, with the right safeguards in place, I could safely and competently care for patients once again. Equally though, they have to safeguard patients and if there was any doubt I would be refused.

The hearing itself was intense. I faced tough questioning from the panel and conflicting opinions from GMC-appointed psychiatrists regarding my readiness to return to work and the risk of relapse. There were moments when I doubted myself and feared the worst. However, I held fast to my conviction that I still had much to contribute as a doctor.

After careful deliberation, the panel ultimately granted me permission to return to practice, although there were strict conditions on my registration. These included close supervision, regular assessments and ongoing monitoring of my mental health. While part of me loathed the restrictions, I understood they were necessary to ensure patient safety and rebuild trust in my abilities.

With a mixture of elation and trepidation, I returned to work at St Mary's Hospital in August 2018, starting all over again almost. I was a clinical observer for eight months (unpaid) and then I had an honorary position that was also unpaid. This was part of a phased return to work. After that, I started at a lower grade of Senior House Officer (the equivalent of Specialty Training 1) for three months. I left St Mary's to go to Charing Cross in Hammersmith for 18 months. Next, I had a post at Barnet Hospital's ICU for six months again covering material I had already covered. I was now convinced that the CSER pathway was too riddled with issues to be worthwhile but I carried on. After a fiercely competitive application process, I was finally accepted onto a Specialty Training 1 post as part of the Acute Care Common Stem programme in North Wales. This was another low as I was effectively going backwards but at least I was now in formal training. I was protected and supported and I was determined to be a doctor again even if it meant starting over.

It was humbling to be told how to complete procedures I had done countless times before. However, I recognised the importance of humility and incremental progress on my journey back to full practice. It was a tough, tough lesson to learn but it has given me a new outlook on life.

I continued to receive support from colleagues and supervisors who recognised my potential. This meant so much to me. They provided opportunities for growth and development, trusting me with greater responsibility as I demonstrated competence and reliability. Slowly but surely, I created a track record that allowed me to manage my own patient caseload once again.

Balancing work with my ongoing mental health needs required vigilance and self-care. I had now found the right medication that did not cause drowsiness (a combination of amisulpride and aripiprazole) and it was life-changing. I maintained open communication with my supervisors and the GMC about how I was doing. My life really was an open book to those that needed access. Over time, I have developed greater self-awareness and resilience, learning to recognise early warning signs of stress and taking proactive steps to manage my well-being.

In June 2021, I officially got my life back. The GMC's conditions on my medical registration and licence were dropped. I was free to practice medicine again without supervision and I want anyone out there in a similar situation to know that it is possible. Obviously, it is not easy, but it is possible to have a mental health episode and to live with a complex condition and be a doctor. I do it every day.

In August 2022, I was enormously proud to accept an offer to enter formal UK medical training at Speciality Training 4 at Darent Valley Hospital. I was happy to be back in my old stomping ground and delighted to have some of my previous examinations and competencies credited to the extent that I could be eligible for this level of training. It really was a special and emotional day.

CHAPTER 8: EMBRACING NEW CHALLENGES—THE PHD JOURNEY

Once I had my life and work on track following my return to medical practice, I decided to pursue a PhD in emergency medicine. Years earlier, Professor Mervyn Singer had inspired me with his passion for research and its potential to improve patient care. Now, feeling stable and purposeful, I felt ready to take on the challenge of doctoral studies, despite the demands it would place on me to balance research with clinical practice.

I reached out to Professor Singer for guidance. He enthusiastically supported my plans and connected me with Professor Karim Brohi, a trauma surgeon and researcher at Queen Mary University of London and the Royal London Hospital. Professor Brohi shared my interest in improving outcomes for critically injured patients and had established the Centre for Trauma Sciences (C4TS) at Queen Mary, bringing together a multidisciplinary research team.

Under Professor Brohi's guidance, I developed a research proposal focused on optimising oxygen delivery for bleeding trauma patients through early intervention and management strategies to improve survival and long-term outcomes. I was excited to combine clinical practice with rigorous scientific inquiry and make a real difference for vulnerable patients.

Securing a place in the PhD program at Queen Mary was thrilling. The C4TS office, filled with brilliant minds and advanced research facilities, was relaxed and organised and so unlike the emergency department. I felt a strong sense of belonging and purpose even though the environment was so different.

I was part of a team of clinical research fellows and managed the day-to-day running of the Centre for Trauma Sciences' trials such as the SWIFT (Study of Whole Blood in Frontline Trauma) trial, the REWIRE (Rescue With Regadenoson) trial and the platform research study ACITII (Activation of Coagulation and Inflammation in Trauma-2) which had been running since 2008. My day-to-day activities included data capture for the participants of our research studies, obtaining consent, attending trauma calls to recruit patients for our trials and running blood samples in our research lab. In short, I was busy, I was learning and I was back with my colleagues. I was Daniel again.

I needed to spend time considering this lifestyle and I prioritised impactful tasks and made time for self-care and personal interests to maintain my mental and physical health.

Collaborating with C4TS's diverse research team was deeply rewarding. I worked with scientists and clinical specialists from various disciplines, each offering unique perspectives and skills. I learned a great deal from our discussions and joint projects.

As I progressed through the PhD program, I developed a deeper appreciation for research's role in driving evidence-based practice and policy. Through my projects and engagement with the scientific community, I recognised the critical part clinician-researchers play in bridging theory and practice by grounding research questions and proposed solutions in the realities of patient care and healthcare system needs.

I completed a self-funded Master's degree in Evidence-Based Healthcare at the University of Oxford from 2020 to 2023, before applying for my PhD in January 2024.

This experience further honed my research skills and deepened my appreciation for the vital role of rigorous evidence in shaping clinical practice.

Reflecting on my PhD journey, I'm struck by the immense personal and professional growth that has come with it. Beyond gaining field-specific knowledge and skills, I have developed critical thinking, project management, problem-solving and communication skills that serve me well to this day.

When I complete my PhD, I would like to combine clinical practice, research and teaching to advance my field and impact patients' and their families' lives. I plan to apply my findings to develop improved treatment protocols and care pathways for better critical illness and injury outcomes. I'm also passionate about mentoring the next generation of emergency medicine clinicians and researchers. I know I can offer them unique support and give them my ear when they need it.

Today I am extremely grateful for the incredible support and opportunities I have received from so many colleagues and friends. I'm especially thankful for the Royal College of Emergency Medicine (RCEM) naming me a Doctoral Fellow for 2024-2026 and funding my PhD. This opened up invaluable mentorship and collaboration opportunities.

As an RCEM doctoral fellow, I've been privileged to be mentored by Professor Ed Barnard, Defence Professor of Emergency Medicine. Our budding relationship has already provided much guidance and support. Professor Barnard's insights into emergency medicine, military medicine and academia have broadened my thinking about my work's potential impact and my career's many possible paths. The fellowship has also let me teach and lead educationally, attending workshops and seminars to share my research and practical knowledge with colleagues and trainees nationwide. These rewarding experiences have allowed me to give back to the emergency medicine community, shape the speciality's future, develop effective communication with diverse learners, and inspire and motivate them.

Thinking back, I'm amazed at how far I've come since the dark days of uncertainty and self-doubt following my illness. The journey back to medicine was long and arduous, but through perseverance, hard work, and unwavering support from colleagues, friends and family, I emerged stronger, more resilient, and more dedicated. The PhD has been integral to this transformation, enriching my clinical practice and opening up new career possibilities. It's taught me to embrace challenges, venture outside my comfort zone and tackle the uncertain and daunting head-on.

I'm thrilled about the opportunities ahead to continue my research on improving critical illness and injury outcomes, apply my findings to shape policy and practice, and supportively mentor the next generation of emergency clinicians and researchers as they navigate this incredible field's challenges and rewards. Above all, I'm grateful for the daily privilege of being an emergency physician and making a difference for patients and families in their most vulnerable moments. I'll never take that privilege for granted and will always strive to provide the highest quality care.

CHAPTER 9: REFLECTIONS AND FUTURE ASPIRATIONS

My path in medicine has been far from conventional, marked by triumphs and tribulations that have shaped me into the physician and person I am today. Through it all, I have learned a great deal about myself and invaluable lessons about my limits too. I value the power of mentorship, the importance of mental health and the unwavering strength of the human spirit more than ever.

The role of mentorship in my personal and professional development cannot be overstated. From the earliest days of my career in the UK, I was fortunate to encounter individuals who saw my potential and were willing to invest their time and expertise in nurturing it. I think back to Mr Kika, the Nigerian consultant at Darent Valley Hospital, who understood the apprehension and challenges I faced as a newcomer to the UK healthcare system. His cultural understanding and willingness to take me under his wing provided a crucial foundation for my integration into the NHS.

Similarly, Mr Witt at UCLH left an indelible mark on my development as a young doctor. I vividly recall his expertise and dedication in his specific field, which was so renowned that patients were referred to him from all over the UK. His mastery was inspiring, showing me the value of focused excellence and continuous improvement in one's craft.

However, it was perhaps Professor Mervyn Singer who had the most profound impact on my career trajectory. During my rotation in the ICU at UCLH, I encountered in him everything I aspired to be as a doctor. His approach to patient care, teaching and research resonated deeply with me. He was not only knowledgeable but also dedicated to our learning, constantly engaging us with questions and ensuring we were absorbing knowledge even as we worked.

Professor Singer's influence extended beyond clinical skills —he was the first to plant the seed of pursuing a PhD and becoming an expert in a particular field. This interaction was transformative, shaping my long-term career aspirations. It was during this time that I made up my mind to become a professor and pursue a PhD, inspired by his example.

The mentorship of Dr Ruth Brown, while initially challenging, proved to be another crucial relationship in my professional development. Her rigorous approach to patient safety and commitment to excellence pushed me to grow and improve constantly. She had a meticulous way of reviewing our work, examining our patient notes and evaluating our decision-making speed and efficiency. While initially intimidating, Dr Brown's mentorship style ultimately fostered a deep respect for patient safety and quality of care that has remained with me throughout my career. Her support during my struggles with mental health also demonstrated the importance of compassionate leadership in medicine.

These mentors, along with many others, have not only shaped my clinical skills but also instilled in me a deep commitment to lifelong learning and the desire to pay it forward by mentoring the next generation of doctors. Their influence has been a guiding light, especially during the darkest periods of my journey.

The unwavering support of my family, friends and colleagues has been a constant source of strength throughout my journey. During my struggles with mental health and the subsequent challenges of rebuilding my career, their encouragement and understanding were invaluable. My sister, in particular, played a crucial role in ensuring I received the help I needed during my first episode. Her persistence in seeking help for me in June 2015 was a pivotal moment that set me on the path to recovery.

I am also deeply grateful for the kindness of strangers who touched my life during difficult times. I vividly remember an encounter with a woman assessing my application for benefits after my bankruptcy—a claim that was ultimately denied. As I shared my story with her, I saw tears welling up in her eyes. Her empathy, even in the face of having to deny my claim, was deeply moving. This moment of human connection amid bureaucratic processes reminded me of the importance of compassion in all aspects of life, including healthcare. If I ever saw her again, I would thank her for her kindness and her humanity.

My journey through mental health challenges has profoundly impacted my personal and professional identity. The experience of living with paranoid schizophrenia, navigating the healthcare system as a patient and rebuilding my career has given me a unique perspective that informs my approach to patient care and my views on the medical profession as a whole.

One of the most significant lessons I've learned is the importance of medication adherence and the transformative power of proper treatment. I vividly recall the moment of clarity that came just four days after starting a new medication regimen during my second hospitalisation. It was as if a fog had lifted, and I suddenly realised the disconnect between my thoughts and reality. This experience has made me a strong advocate for mental health treatment and has given me a deep empathy for patients struggling with their own mental health challenges.

The stigma surrounding mental health in the medical profession became painfully clear to me during my recovery. I encountered well-meaning colleagues who wanted to guide me through alternative career paths. They thought they were being helpful but there is an endemic misunderstanding of mental health conditions in high-stress careers. One particularly poignant memory stands out when a clinical director at UCLH suggested I consider an alternative speciality upon learning of my diagnosis. There was a dominant stigma that patients could not recover. Now it makes me wonder how many medics have quietly abandoned their careers believing they were no longer competent.

These experiences have fuelled my determination to challenge that stigma in medicine. I believe that by sharing my story openly, I can help break down barriers and foster a more supportive environment for healthcare professionals facing similar challenges.

The importance of being self-aware, vulnerable and speaking openly when addressing mental health challenges cannot be overstated. Throughout my recovery and return to practice, I've learned the value of being honest about my experiences and needs. This openness has not only aided my own healing but has also created opportunities for meaningful conversations with colleagues and mentors.

My journey can serve as a powerful tool for advocacy and education. By speaking plainly about what has happened to me, I hope to encourage others to seek help when needed and to challenge the idea that mental health struggles are incompatible with a successful medical career. There is too much secrecy and I am more convinced than ever of the need for greater support, resources and understanding for healthcare workers facing mental health challenges.

The culture of medicine focuses on being resilient and self-reliant but those qualities at work can sometimes create barriers to seeking help. I would prefer to see a shift towards a culture of support, where vulnerability is seen as a strength rather than a weakness. This includes creating more accessible pathways for mental health support, reducing stigma through education and having safe and open dialogue. The NHS policies that are associated with staff with mental health issues need to protect the careers of those who seek help. In turn that would put patient safety at the forefront as well as support vulnerable people who are scared that they will lose their livelihood.

One of the hardest times I have endured was not being sectioned or spending time in mental health units—it was rebuilding my career after my illness. Returning to practice at a lower level than I had previously achieved was especially hard for me. I had to find the motivation every day to show up and work, knowing I was capable of more. This constant need for self-motivation was perhaps the hardest part of the entire experience.

However, this experience also taught me the value of focusing on long-term goals (even when I was trying to live one day at a time). I learned to find meaning and purpose in each day I was learning skills that I had already mastered; on days when progress seemed slow. This mindset has been crucial in sustaining my motivation and drive throughout my career recovery. I've come to see each challenge as an opportunity for growth and each setback as a chance to refine my skills and knowledge. This attitude helped me when I had to start all over again in medicine and had a mountain to climb.

Now, I have a lot to look forward to—my short-term goals include completing my PhD in Trauma Sciences and obtaining a consultant position in emergency medicine. These milestones represent not just personal achievements, but opportunities to contribute more significantly to the field of emergency medicine and to mentor the next generation of doctors.

My long-term aspirations extend beyond clinical practice. I aim to become a respected leader and innovator within emergency medicine, contributing to advancements in patient care, research and medical education. I envision myself in a role where I can influence policy, drive innovation, and shape the future of emergency care but I do not want to forget what has happened. Amongst these plans, I will serve as a mentor and role model for emerging emergency physicians. I want to offer them the kind of supportive, nurturing environment that was so crucial in my own development. I aim to foster a culture of inclusivity, support and collaboration, where diverse perspectives are valued and all members of the healthcare team can thrive. I am determined to use my story to inspire hope and make change.

Throughout this journey, I've come to appreciate the critical importance of work-life balance and self-care in sustaining a fulfilling career in medicine. The demands of emergency medicine are intense, and I've learned that maintaining my own well-being is not just a personal necessity but a professional responsibility. I strive to model healthy work-life balance for my colleagues and mentees, emphasising the importance of self-care, maintaining strong support networks and pursuing interests outside of medicine.

As I reflect on my journey, I am filled with gratitude for the opportunities, experiences and lessons I've gained. Every challenge, every setback and every triumph has contributed to my growth and development as a person and as a physician, even if it did not feel that way at the time. I am thankful for the patients who have trusted me with their care, the colleagues who have supported and challenged me, and the mentors who have guided my path.

'The business of life is the acquisition of memories.' I cannot remember where this quote came from but those words have guided me through difficult times. They helped me so much. I used to say them out loud to myself when I could not understand why my life was so full of challenges.

It is important to say at this point that my journey is far from over. I still have hard days. I still have goals that have been delayed by years of difficulties. But I face the future with optimism, armed with the lessons of the past and supported by the incredible network of family, friends and colleagues who have been by my side. As I continue to grow as a physician, researcher and leader, I remain committed to the core values that have guided me: compassion, excellence, resilience and an unwavering dedication to improving the lives of others.

The road ahead may not always be smooth, but I am ready to embrace whatever comes my way. For in each challenge lies an opportunity for growth, in each setback a chance for learning, and in each triumph a moment to inspire others. As I step forward into this next chapter of my career, I do so with gratitude for the past, enthusiasm for the present, and hope for the future. The journey continues, and I am excited to see where it will lead.

CHAPTER 10: FINAL WORDS

I wasn't fully prepared for the setbacks I've experienced, but I found I could draw on the skills I had developed in pursuing my goals. The determination and focus that had helped me succeed in medical school and my early career became the same qualities that saw me through my recovery and the rebuilding of my professional life. I am grateful for the hardworking ethos my parents modelled for us as children. I used their example to work hard at recovering my mental health.

One key strategy I've employed is what I call the 'bite-sized' approach to advancing my career. This method has been instrumental in helping me navigate complex challenges and achieve my goals. The process involves identifying my ultimate goal, meticulously plotting out a route to get there, and then following that route with unwavering focus and determination.

This approach served me well during my recovery and subsequent professional rebuilding. When faced with the daunting task of returning to medicine after my illness, I broke down the process into smaller, manageable steps. First, stabilising my mental health and adhering to my treatment plan. Then, rebuilding my knowledge base and clinical skills. Next, gaining practical experience, even if it meant starting at a lower level than before.

Each of these steps, while challenging, felt achievable when viewed as part of a larger plan. This 'bite-sized' approach allowed me to maintain my focus and motivation, even when progress seemed slow. It gave me a sense of accomplishment with each small goal achieved, which in turn fuelled my determination to keep pushing forward.

The transformative power of resilience, perseverance and self-belief has shaped my values and deepened my passion for medicine. These qualities have taught me that setbacks, no matter how severe, are not the end of the story but rather pivotal moments that can lead to growth and new opportunities.

My experiences have reinforced the importance of staying true to one's values and passions, even in the face of adversity. There were moments when it would have been easier to give up on medicine, to accept the limitations that others tried to place on me because of my diagnosis. However, my passion for emergency medicine and my desire to help others were too strong to be extinguished by these challenges. In short, if you are following your heart's desire you need to find a way to keep going.

One of the most profound lessons I've learned is the importance of living in the present and valuing the people who are with you right now. Life is unpredictable, and circumstances can change in an instant. I didn't have the time with my dad that I would have liked so I now try to make the most of every moment and every interaction, and that means learning to switch off from stress and learning to relax.

This philosophy influences both my personal life and my medical practice. In my personal life, I really cherish the time I spend with family and friends. I make sure I tell them I appreciate their support and that I care about them. In my medical practice, this belief has enhanced my ability to connect with patients and provide compassionate care.

As I look towards the future, I am committed to using my experiences to inspire and empower others who may be facing similar challenges. I want my story to be a source of hope for those who are struggling, a reminder that setbacks—even serious ones like mental health diagnoses—do not have to be the end of one's dreams. I want to challenge the stigma surrounding mental health in the medical profession and advocate for a more compassionate, inclusive approach to supporting healthcare workers who are facing personal struggles.

To those who are in the midst of their own challenges, remember that you are stronger than you know. The qualities that have brought you this far—your perseverance, your resilience, your self-belief—are still within you, even if they feel distant right now. Don't be afraid to seek help and support, even if you have to ask again and again.

To my colleagues in the medical profession, I urge you to be kind to yourselves and to each other. The demands of our profession are intense, and it's easy to become overwhelmed or to neglect our own well-being in the service of others. Taking care of our mental and physical health is essential for providing the best care to our patients and for sustaining fulfilling careers in medicine.

As I continue on my own journey, I remain committed to my core values of compassion, excellence and continuous growth. I am excited about the future and I know there will be good times and bad but it is my journey and I have good coping mechanisms and I know how to seek support.

In closing, I want to emphasise that our journeys are never truly complete. There will always be new challenges to face, new goals to strive for, and new opportunities for growth and learning. But armed with perseverance, resilience and self-belief, we can face whatever comes our way with courage and determination.

To those reading my story, I hope you find within it something that resonates with your own experiences, something that inspires you to keep pushing forward in the face of adversity, something that reminds you of your own strength and resilience. Remember, your story is still being written. Make it one that fills you with pride, one that inspires others, one that leaves the world a little better than you found it.

Story Terrace

Printed in Great Britain
by Amazon

74b60a6d-ce96-4b5b-aab1-15b117673a7bR01